Alkaline Diet for Busy People

A Collection of Cheap and Tasty Alkaline Recipes to Save
Your Money and Satisfy Your Taste

Gerard Short

Table of Contents

MORNING SOUFFLE

Serves: *4*

Prep Time: *15* Minutes

Cook Time: *35* Minutes

Total Time: *50* Minutes

INGREDIENTS

- ¼ cup green chilies
- 1 cup avocado
- 1 cup grilled chicken
- 2 onions
- 4 eggs
- ½ cup milk
- 1 tablespoon coconut flour
- 1 tsp salt
- ¼ tsp pepper

DIRECTIONS

1. Scatter green chillies in the bottom of a baking dish

2. Add chicken, onions, avocado over green chillies and set aside

3. In another bowl combine coconut flour with eggs, pepper, salt and pour egg mixture over vegetables

4. Bake at 350 F for 30-35 minutes

5. When ready garnish with cilantro and serve

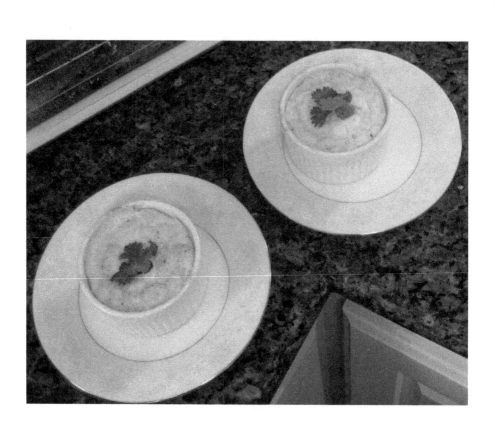

BUCKWHEAT MUFFINS

Serves: 8-12

Prep Time: 10   Minutes

Cook Time: 15   Minutes

Total Time: 25   Minutes

INGREDIENTS

-        1 cup buckwheat groats

-        ½ cup coconut flakes

-        ¼ cup walnuts

-        ¼ cup pumpkin seeds

-        1 tablespoon chia seeds

-        ¼ cup flaxseed meal

-        1 tsp cinnamon

-        2 eggs

-        1 cup almond milk

-        ¼ cup almond butter

-        2 packets powdered stevia

-        1 tablespoon vanilla extract

DIRECTIONS

1. In a bowl soak buckwheat groats overnight

2. In a bowl combine pumpkin seeds, buckwheat groats, chia seeds, cinnamon, salt, walnuts, flaxseed meal and coconut flakes

3. In a bowl combine almond milk, powdered stevia, eggs and combine

4. Combine almond mix mixture with buckwheat mixture and pour mixture into 8-12 muffins cups

5. Bake at 350 F for 12-15 minutes

6. When ready remove from the oven and serve

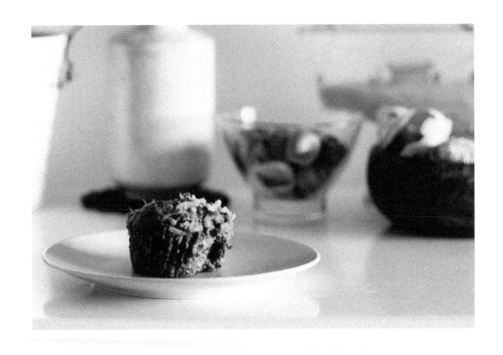

MUSHROOM OMELETTE

Serves: *1*

Prep Time: *5*   Minutes

Cook Time: *10*   Minutes

Total Time: *15*   Minutes

INGREDIENTS

-        2 eggs

-        ¼ tsp salt

-        ¼ tsp black pepper

-        1 tablespoon olive oil

-        ¼ cup cheese

-        ¼ tsp basil

-        1 cup mushrooms

DIRECTIONS

1. In a bowl combine all ingredients together and mix well

2. In a skillet heat olive oil and pour the egg mixture

3. Cook for 1-2 minutes per side

4. When ready remove omelette from the skillet and serve

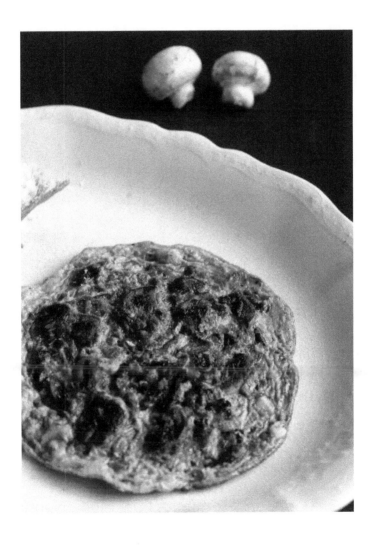

FRENCH TOAST

Serves: *4*

Prep Time: *10*   Minutes

Cook Time: *20*   Minutes

Total Time: *30*   Minutes

INGREDIENTS

-         5 egg whites

-         ½ cup low fat milk

-         ¼ tsp cinnamon

-         ½ tsp allspice

-         4 slices bread

-         1 tsp butter

DIRECTIONS

1. In a bowl mix egg whites, cinnamon, allspice and milk

2. Dip bread into batter and place in a skillet

3. Cook for 1-2 minutes per side or until golden

4. When ready, remove and serve

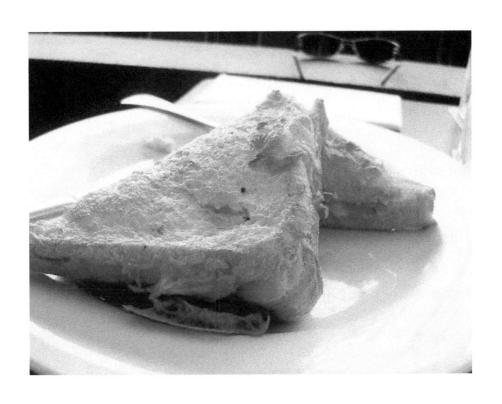

ORANGE MORNING COFFE

Serves: 2

Prep Time: 5 Minutes

Cook Time: 5 Minutes

Total Time: 10 Minutes

INGREDIENTS

- ½ cup instant coffee

- ¾ cup sugar

- 1 cup Coffee Mate powder

- 1 tsp dried orange peel

DIRECTIONS

1. Place all ingredients in a blender and blend until powdered

2. Place 2 tsp of coffee mix in a cup

3. Add boiling water and mix, serve when ready

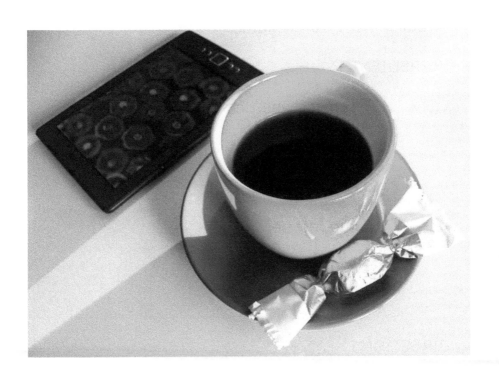

MORNING FRUIT COMPOTE

Serves: *1*

Prep Time: *10*   Minutes

Cook Time: *10*   Minutes

Total Time: *20*   Minutes

INGREDIENTS

-        ½ cup strawberries

-        ¼ cup blackberries

-        ¼ cup peaches

-        ½ cup raspberries

-        ¼ cup orange juice

-        1 banana

DIRECTIONS

1. Pour orange juice into a container

2. Add remaining ingredients and toss well

3. Allow to rest overnight

4. Serve when ready

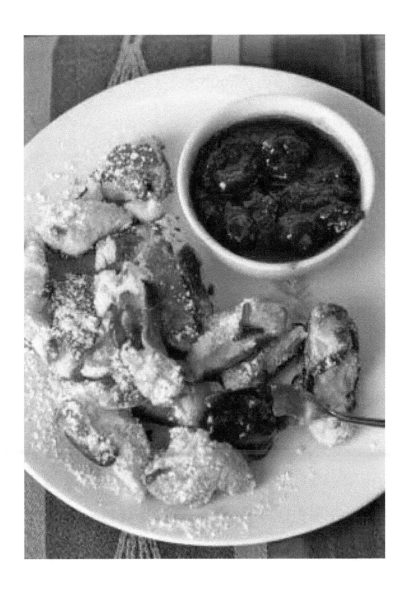

BAKED EGG CUSTARD

Serves: *4*

Prep Time: *10*   Minutes

Cook Time: *30*   Minutes

Total Time: *40*   Minutes

INGREDIENTS

-        2 eggs

-        ½ cup low fat milk

-        2 tablespoons sugar

-        1 tsp vanilla

-        1 tsp nutmeg

DIRECTIONS

1. Preheat the oven to 300 F

2. In a bowl mix all ingredients using a hand mixer

3. Pour into muffin pans and sprinkle nutmeg

4. Bake for 25-30 minutes

5. When ready remove and serve

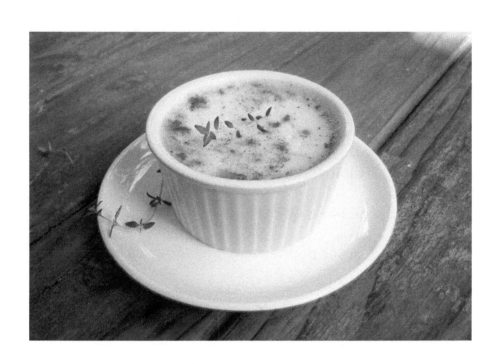

EGG OMELET

Serves: *4*

Prep Time: *5* minutes

Cook Time: *10* minutes

Total Time: *15* minutes

INGREDIENTS

- 3 eggs beaten

- 3 tablespoons 2% milk

- 2 teaspoons butter

- dash of pepper

DIRECTIONS

1. Beat eggs with milk and pepper

2. Heat butter in skillet and add eggs

3. When eggs are done roll one half over

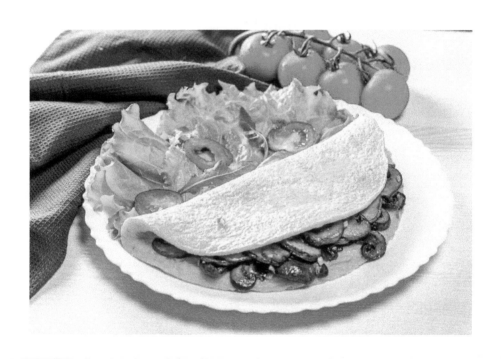

GREEN CHILI CHEESE OMELETE

Serves: *4*

Prep Time: *15*   minutes

Cook Time: *0*   minutes

Total Time: *15*   minutes

INGREDIENTS

-        1 tablespoon butter

-        4 eggs

-        4 tablespoons water

-        1 4-ounce can green chilies

-        4 oz. cheese

Sauce

-        1 tablespoon butter

-        1 tablespoon onion

-        ¼ cup canned tomatoes

DIRECTIONS

1. Beat eggs and water together, meanwhile melt butter in skillet

2. Add egg mixture and reduce heat

3. Wrap chilies around each cheese strips

4. Serve on heated platter

5. For sauce melt butter and add tomato and onion

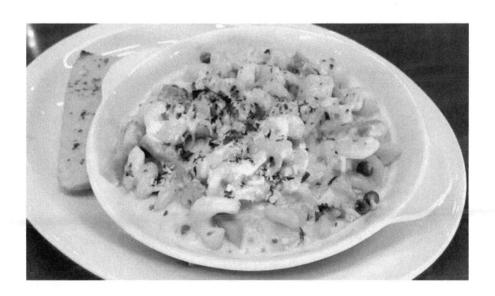

MACARONI AND CHEESE

Serves: *4*

Prep Time: *15*   minutes

Cook Time: *20*   minutes

Total Time: *35*   minutes

INGREDIENTS

-        8 oz. macaroni

-        1 tablespoon canola oil

-        2 teaspoons chives

-        ¾ teaspoon pepper

-        1 ½ cups natural cheese

-        ½ cup 1,5% milk

DIRECTIONS

1. Heat 5-6 cups of water and add macaroni for about 8-10 minutes

2. Drain and rinse in cold water

3. Add canola oil and stir until macaroni is coated

4. Add milk, cheese, pepper and chives

5. Mix in cheese with macaroni and reduce heat

6. Continue cooking for 15-20 minutes

7. Add 1-2 tablespoons of milk

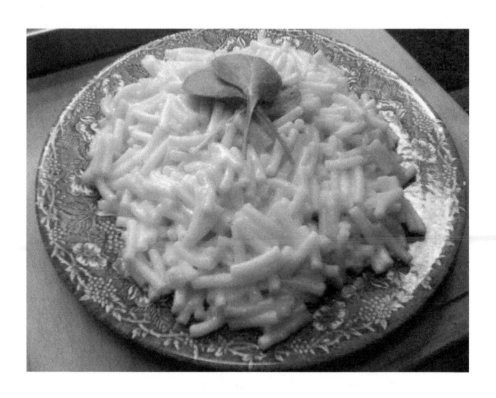

CREPES

Serves: 6

Prep Time: 10 minutes

Cook Time: 10 minutes

Total Time: 20 minutes

INGREDIENTS

- 3 eggs

- 1 ¼ cups 1,5% milk

- ¾ cup sifted flour

- 1 tablespoon sugar

- ¼ teaspoon salt

- cooking spray

DIRECTIONS

1. Beat eggs until thick

2. Add salt and sugar

3. Add flour with milk beating with mixer

4. Spread batter evenly to make thin cakes

5. Turn when is brown

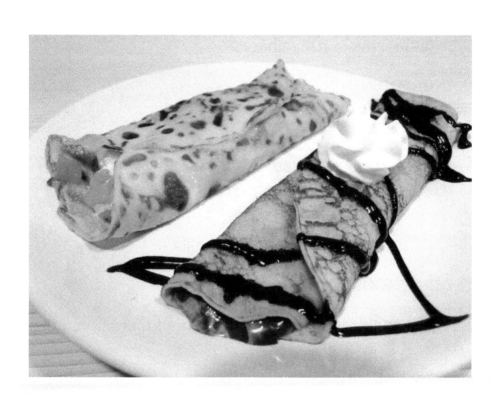

GRILLED CHEESE SANDWICH

Serves: 4

Prep Time: 20   minutes

Cook Time: 0   minutes

Total Time: 20   minutes

INGREDIENTS

-        2 tablespoons butter

-        8 slices bread

-        8 oz. Swiss cheese

-        1 4-ounce can green chills

DIRECTIONS

1. Spread butter on the side of four slices of bread

2. Place 1 ounce of Swiss cheese and one whole chili

3. Place cheese on split chili and top with remaining slice of bread

4. Heat skillet and place sandwiches in skillet

5. Grill on each side until cheese is melted

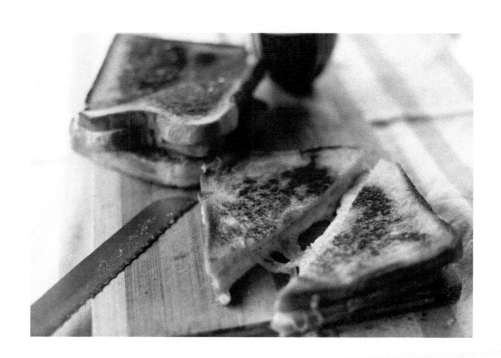

CINNAMON FRENCH TOAST

Serves: 4

Prep Time: 5 minutes

Cook Time: 10 minutes

Total Time: 15 minutes

INGREDIENTS

- 2 eggs

- 1-2 tablespoons butter

- cinnamon

- ¾ cup light non-diary creamer

- 6 slices bread

DIRECTIONS

1. Combine eggs and creamer

2. Dup bread in egg mixture

3. Melt one tablespoon of butter

4. Sprinkle top side with cinnamon

5. If needed add more butter

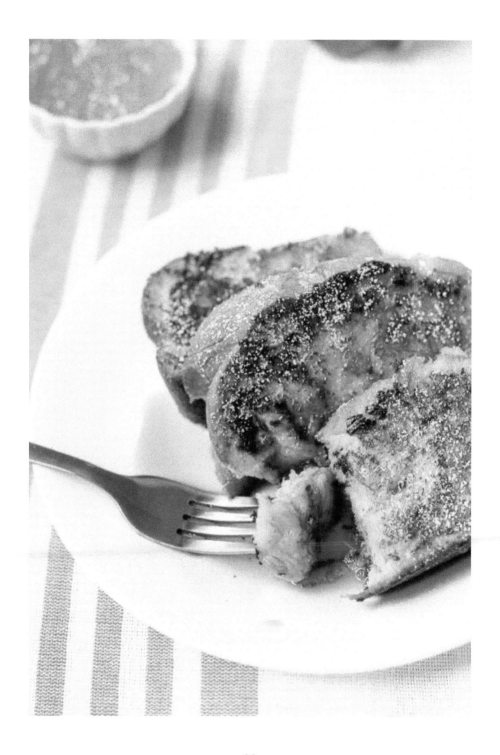

BANANA PANCAKES

Serves: *4*

Prep Time: *10* Minutes

Cook Time: *20* Minutes

Total Time: *30* Minutes

INGREDIENTS

-        1 cup whole wheat flour

-        ¼ tsp baking soda

-        ¼ tsp baking powder

-        1 cup mashed banana

-         2 eggs

-        1 cup milk

DIRECTIONS

1. In a bowl combine all ingredients together and mix well

2. In a skillet heat olive oil

3. Pour ¼ of the batter and cook each pancake for 1-2 minutes per side

4. When ready remove from heat and serve

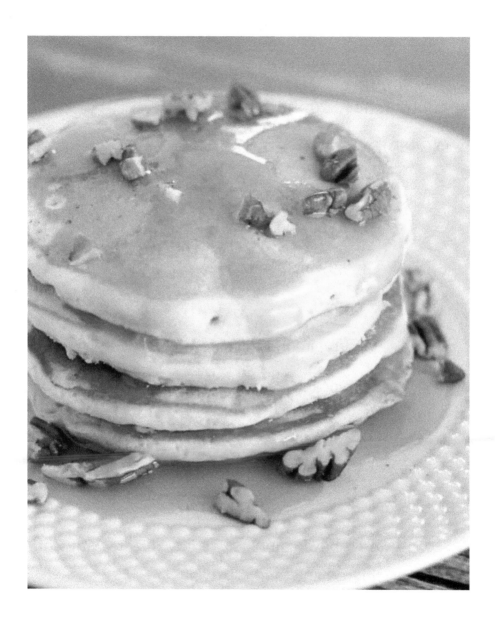

AVOCADO PANCAKES

Serves: 4

Prep Time: 5   Minutes

Cook Time: 15   Minutes

Total Time: 20   Minutes

INGREDIENTS

- ¼ cup coconut flour

- ¼ tsp baking soda

- ¼ tsp salt

- 2 eggs

- ¼ cup almond milk

- ¼ avocado

- 2 green onions

- 1 tablespoon olive oil

DIRECTIONS

1. In a bowl combine dry ingredients with wet ingredients and mix well

2. In a skillet heat olive oil and pour ¼ batter and cook for 1-2 minutes per side

3. When ready remove to a place and serve with avocado slices

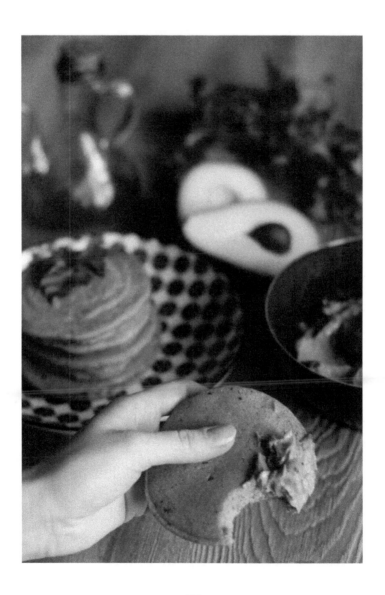

OLD FASHIONED PANCAKES

Serves: *4*

Prep Time: *10*   Minutes

Cook Time: *20*   Minutes

Total Time: *30*   Minutes

INGREDIENTS

- 1 egg

- ½ cup sugar

- ½ tsp baking powder

- ½ cup low fat milk

- 1 tsp vegetable oil

- ½ cup all purpose flour

DIRECTIONS

1. In a bowl mix all purpose flour, egg, sugar, baking powder, milk and water

2. Pour ¼ cup batter in a skillet and cook for 1-2 minutes per side

3. When ready remove and serve

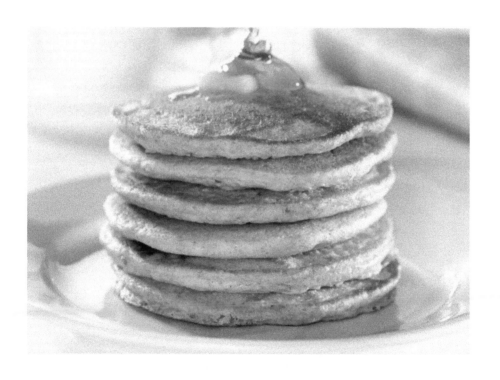

BREAKFAST COOKIES

Serves: 8-12

Prep Time: 5 Minutes

Cook Time: 15 Minutes

Total Time: 20 Minutes

INGREDIENTS

- 1 cup rolled oats

- ¼ cup applesauce

- ½ tsp vanilla extract

- 3 tablespoons chocolate chips

- 2 tablespoons dried fruits

- 1 tsp cinnamon

DIRECTIONS

1. Preheat the oven to 325 F

2. In a bowl combine all ingredients together and mix well

3. Scoop cookies using an ice cream scoop

4. Place cookies onto a prepared baking sheet

5. Place in the oven for 12-15 minutes or until the cookies are done

6. When ready remove from the oven and serve

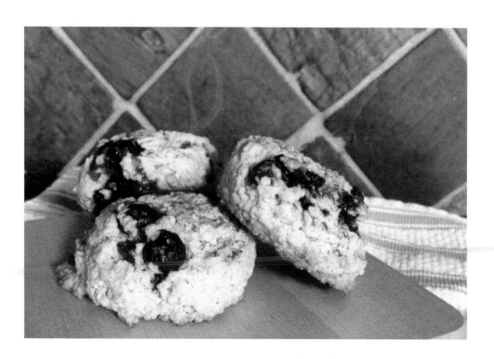

PINEAPPLE PUDDING

Serves: *4*

Prep Time: *10*   Minutes

Cook Time: *20*   Minutes

Total Time: *30*   Minutes

INGREDIENTS

- 2 tablespoons all-purpose flour

- ½ cup sugar

- 1 egg

- 2 eggs

- 1 cup low fat milk

- 1 cup water

- 1 tsp vanilla extract

- 1 cup pineapple chunks

- ½ cup sugar

- 24-26 vanilla wafers

DIRECTIONS

1. Preheat the oven to 400 F

2. In a saucepan add sugar, egg, flour, egg yolks

3. Stir in water, milk and cook until water boils

4. Remove from heat, add vanilla extract and spread 1 tablespoon on the bottom of a casserole dish

5. Top with vanilla wafer and pineapples, continue with layers of custard, vanilla and wafers

6. Beat remaining egg whites using a hand mixer

7. Pile beaten egg whites on top of layered pudding

8. Bake for 8-10 minutes

9. Remove and serve

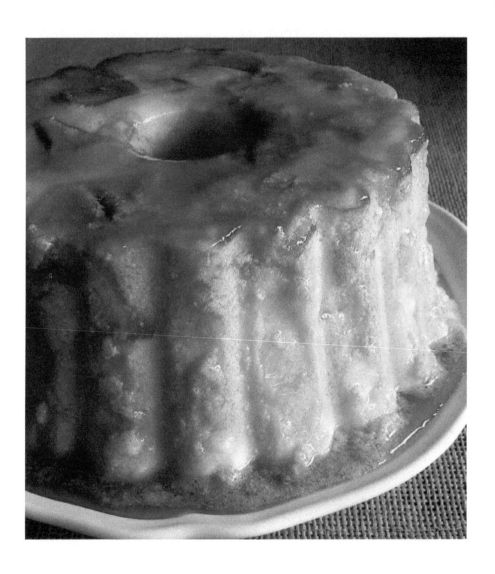

JEWELED COOKIES

Serves: *12*

Prep Time: *10*   Minutes

Cook Time: *15*   Minutes

Total Time: *25*   Minutes

INGREDIENTS

-        1 cup brown sugar

-        1 egg

-        ½ cup milk

-        ¼ cup unsalted butter

-        1 tsp vanilla

-        1 cup all-purpose flour

-        1 tsp baking powder

-        12 gumdrops

DIRECTIONS

1. Preheat the oven to 375 F

2. Cream butter, egg and sugar

3. Stir in vanilla and milk

4. In a bowl mix flour with baking powder and add remaining ingredients

5. Mix well and let it rest for 50-60 minutes

6. Drop dough onto cookie sheet

7. Bake for 10-12 minutes or until golden brown

8. Remove and serve

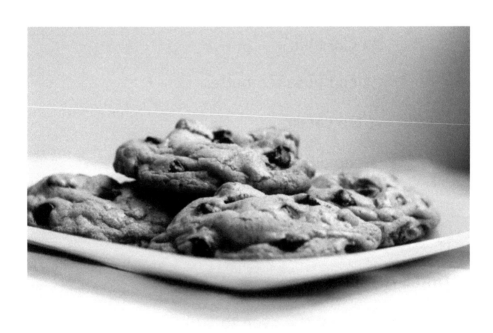

PUMPKIN SOUFFLE

Serves: *1*

Prep Time: *10* Minutes

Cook Time: *45* Minutes

Total Time: *55* Minutes

INGREDIENTS

- ¼ cup apple juice concentrate

- 1 can pumpkin

- 1 cup milk

- ¼ cup water

- ¼ tsp vanilla extract

- ¼ tsp ground nutmeg

- ¼ tsp all spice

- 1 tsp cinnamon

- ¼ cup grape nuts

- ¼ tsp pumpkin pie spice

DIRECTIONS

1. Preheat the oven to 375 F

2. In a bowl add all ingredients except grape nuts

3. In a pie plate add mixture and sprinkle grape nuts

4. Bake for 40-45 minutes, serve when ready

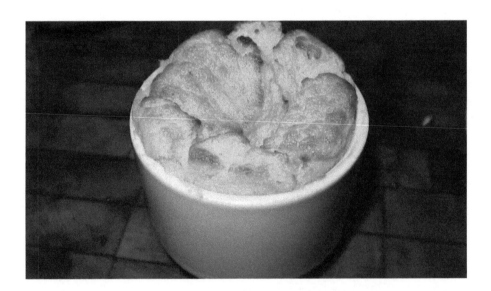

POUND CAKE

Serves: *4*

Prep Time: *10* Minutes

Cook Time: *30* Minutes

Total Time: *40* Minutes

INGREDIENTS

- ½ lb. butter

- ¾ cup sugar

- 3 eggs

- 1,5 cup bread flour

- 4 oz. milk

DIRECTIONS

1. Preheat the oven to 350 F

2. Cream butter and add sugar

3. Bell well, add flour, milk, eggs and mix

4. Pour batter in a baking dish and bake for 30 minutes

5. When ready remove and serve

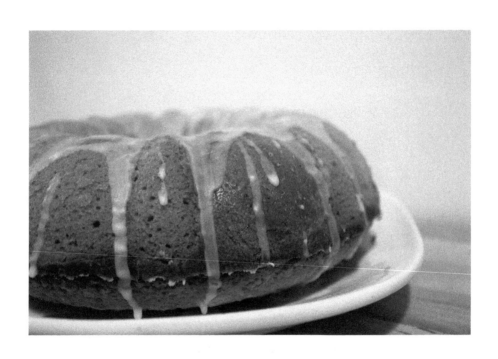

PUMPKIN SMOOTHIE

Serves: *1*

Prep Time: *5* Minutes

Cook Time: *5* Minutes

Total Time: *10* Minutes

INGREDIENTS

- 2 tablespoons pumpkin

- 4 tablespoons coconut milk

- 1 tsp honey

- 1 banana

- ¼ tsp cinnamon

- 1 cup ice

DIRECTIONS

1. In a blender place all ingredients and blend until smooth

2. Pour smoothie in a glass and serve

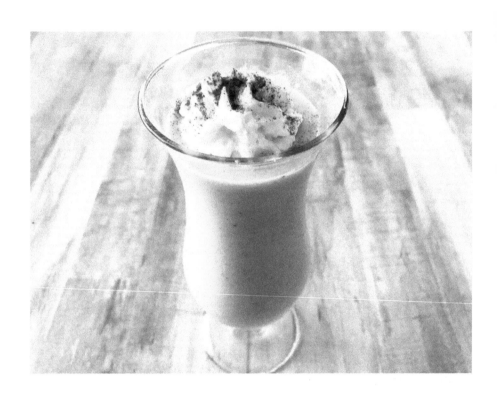

KIWI SMOOTHIE

Serves: *1*

Prep Time: *5*   Minutes

Cook Time: *5*   Minutes

Total Time: *10*   Minutes

INGREDIENTS

-       2 kiwis

-       2 bananas

-       1 cup soy milk

-       1 cup yogurt

-       2 tablespoons porridge oats

-        1 tsp honey

DIRECTIONS

1. In a blender place all ingredients and blend until smooth

2. Pour smoothie in a glass and serve

BERRY KALE SMOOTHIE

Serves: *1*

Prep Time: *5*   Minutes

Cook Time: *5*   Minutes

Total Time: *10* Minutes

INGREDIENTS

-       1 handful kale

-       1 banana

-       1 cup berries

-       1 cup almond milk

-       1 cup protein powder

DIRECTIONS

1. In a blender place all ingredients and blend until smooth

2. Pour smoothie in a glass and serve

COCONUT SMOOTHIE

Serves: *1*

Prep Time: *5*   Minutes

Cook Time: *5*   Minutes

Total Time: *10*   Minutes

INGREDIENTS

-        1 cup coconut milk

-        ½ cup pineapple chunks

-        1 banana

-        ½ cup pineapple juice

-        1 cup ice

DIRECTIONS

1. In a blender place all ingredients and blend until smooth

2. Pour smoothie in a glass and serve

AVOCADO SMOOTHIE

Serves: *1*

Prep Time: *5*   Minutes

Cook Time: *5*   Minutes

Total Time: *10*   Minutes

INGREDIENTS

-        1 cup coconut milk

-        1 cup pineapple chunks

-        1 avocado

-        1 banana

-        1 tsp vanilla extract

-        1 tablespoon hemp seeds

-        1 cup ice

DIRECTIONS

1. In a blender place all ingredients and blend until smooth

2. Pour smoothie in a glass and serve

TURMERIC SMOOTHIE

Serves: 1

Prep Time: 5   Minutes

Cook Time: 5   Minutes

Total Time: 10   Minutes

INGREDIENTS

-        1 banana

-        1 cup almond milk

-        1 tsp turmeric

-        1 tsp ginger

-        1 tsp cinnamon

-        1 tsp honey

-        1 cup ice

DIRECTIONS

1. In a blender place all ingredients and blend until smooth

2. Pour smoothie in a glass and serve

PAPAYA SMOOTHIE

Serves: *1*

Prep Time: *5*   Minutes

Cook Time: *5*   Minutes

Total Time: *10*   Minutes

INGREDIENTS

-        1 banana

-        1 cup papaya

-        1 cup blueberries

-        1 tsp cinnamon

-        1 cup spinach

-        1 tablespoon chia seeds

-        1 cup almond milk

DIRECTIONS

1. In a blender place all ingredients and blend until smooth

2. Pour smoothie in a glass and serve

APPLE SMOOTHIE

Serves: *1*

Prep Time: *5*   Minutes

Cook Time: *5*   Minutes

Total Time: *10*   Minutes

INGREDIENTS

-        1 apple

-        1 cup spinach

-        1 cup kale

-        1 cup ice

DIRECTIONS

1. In a blender place all ingredients and blend until smooth

2. Pour smoothie in a glass and serve

SIMPLE MUFFINS

Serves: *8-12*

Prep Time: *10*   Minutes

Cook Time: *20*   Minutes

Total Time: *30*   Minutes

INGREDIENTS

-          2 eggs

-          1 tablespoon olive oil

-          1 cup milk

-          2 cups whole wheat flour

-          1 tsp baking soda

-          ¼ tsp baking soda

-          1 cup pumpkin puree

-          1 tsp cinnamon

-          ¼ cup molasses

DIRECTIONS

1. In a bowl combine all wet ingredients

2. In another bowl combine all dry ingredients

3. Combine wet and dry ingredients together

4. Pour mixture into 8-12 prepared muffin cups, fill 2/3 of the cups

5. Bake for 18-20 minutes at 375 F

6. When ready remove from the oven and serve

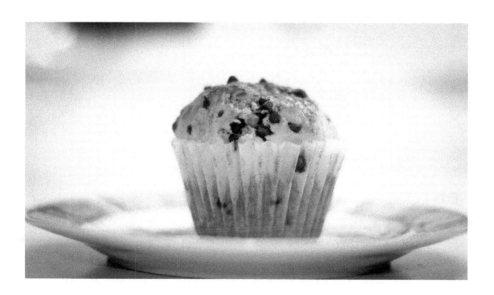

CORN BREAD & MUFFINS

Serves: *8*

Prep Time: *10*   minutes

Cook Time: *25*   minutes

Total Time: *35*   minutes

INGREDIENTS

-        ¾ cup boiling water

-        ¾ cup cornmeal

-        2 eggs

-        1 tablespoon butter

-        1 tablespoon sugar

-        ¼ teaspoon salt

DIRECTIONS

1. Heat oven at 375 degrees

2. Stir boiling water gradually into cornmeal

3. Beat egg whites until stiff and hold in reserve

4. Beat butter, yolks, egg, salt, sugar into cornmeal mixture

5. Bake for 25 minutes

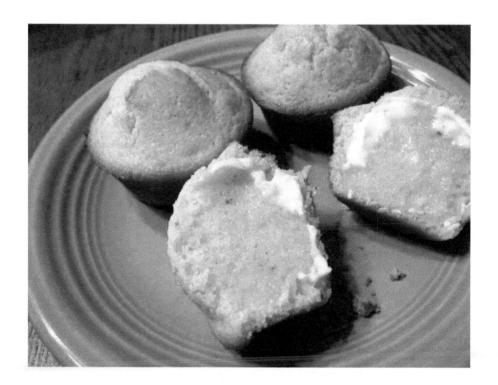

OATMEAL RAISIN MUFFINS

Serves: *4*

Prep Time: *10* minutes

Cook Time: *15* minutes

Total Time: *25* minutes

INGREDIENTS

- 1 cup cake flour

- ½ cup white flour

- 2 teaspoons baking powder

- ¾ cup rolled oats

- ½ cup 1,5% milk

- 1 egg

- 4 tablespoons butter

- 3 tablespoons honey

- ½ cup raisins

- ½ cup water

- 1 ½ teaspoons cinnamon

DIRECTIONS

1. Sift the flour and baking powder

2. Mix in rolled oats and cinnamon

3. Beat egg, milk, butter and honey

4. Add raisins

5. Add the flour mixture and stir until ingredients are blended

6. Bake at 400 degrees for 10-12 minutes

TOMATO WRAP

Serves: *4*

Prep Time: *5*   Minutes

Cook Time: *15*   Minutes

Total Time: *20*   Minutes

INGREDIENTS

-      1 cup corn

-      1 cup tomatoes

-      1 cup pickles

-      1 tablespoon olive oil

-      1 tablespoon mayonnaise

-      6-7 turkey slices

-      2-3 whole-wheat tortillas

-      1 cup romaine lettuce

DIRECTIONS

1. In a bowl combine tomatoes, pickles, olive oil, corn and set aside

2. Place the turkey slices over the tortillas and top with tomato mixture and mayonnaise

3. Roll and serve

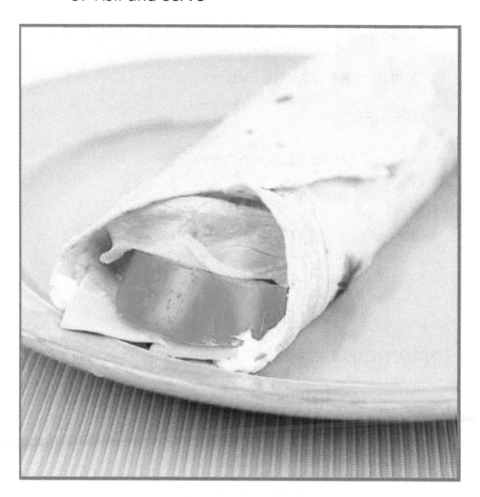

THYME COD

Serves: 2

Prep Time: 5   Minutes

Cook Time: 15   Minutes

Total Time: 20   Minutes

INGREDIENTS

-       1 tablespoon olive oil

-       ½ red onion

-       1 can tomatoes

-       2-3 springs thyme

-       2-3 cod fillets

DIRECTIONS

1. In a frying pan heat olive oil and sauté onion, stir in tomatoes, spring thyme and cook for 5-6 minutes

2. Add cod fillets, cover and cook for 5-6 minutes per side

3. When ready remove from heat and serve

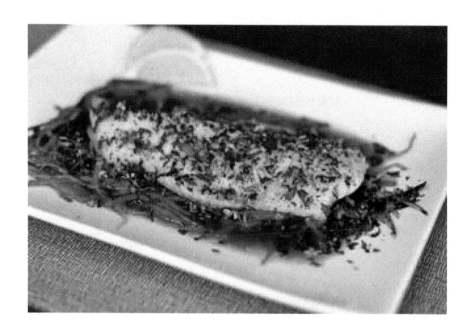

VEGGIE STIR-FRY

Serves: 2

Prep Time: 10 Minutes

Cook Time: 20 Minutes

Total Time: 30 Minutes

INGREDIENTS

- 1 tablespoon cornstarch

- 1 garlic clove

- ¼ cup olive oil

- ¼ head broccoli

- ¼ cup show peas

- ½ cup carrots

- ¼ cup green beans

- 1 tablespoon soy sauce

- ½ cup onion

DIRECTIONS

1. In a bowl combine garlic, olive oil, cornstarch and mix well

2. Add the rest of the ingredients and toss to coat

3. In a skillet cook vegetables mixture until tender

4. When ready transfer to a plate garnish with ginger and serve

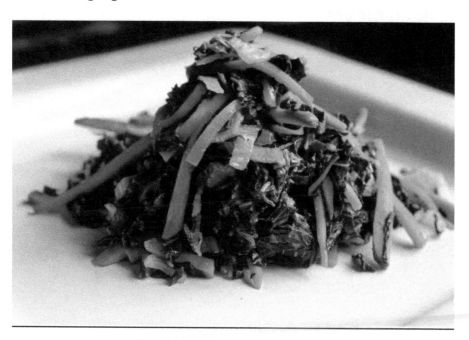

PINEAPPLE-MANGO SMOOTHIE

Serves: *1*

Prep Time: *5* Minutes

Cook Time: *5* Minutes

Total Time: *10* Minutes

INGREDIENTS

- 1 tsp vanilla powder

- 1 mango

- 1 cup baby spinach

- 1 cup ice

DIRECTIONS

1. In a blender place all ingredients and blend until smooth

2. Pour smoothie in a glass and serve

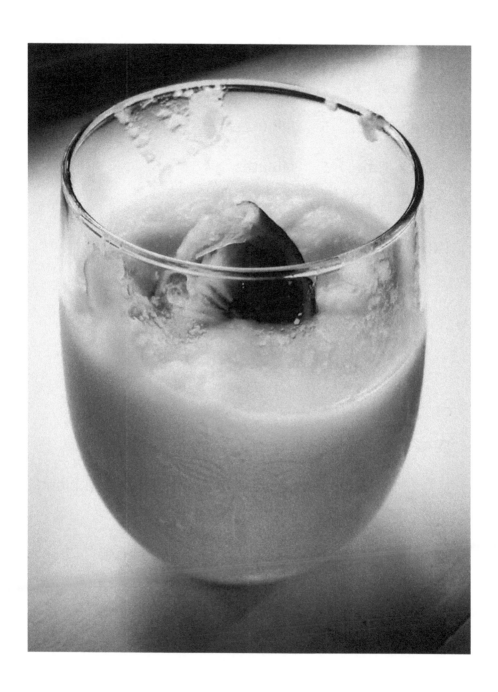

ALMOND-BANANA SMOOTHIE

Serves: 1

Prep Time: 5   Minutes

Cook Time: 5   Minutes

Total Time: 10   Minutes

INGREDIENTS

-       1 banana

-       1 cup almond milk

-       ¼ tsp vanilla extract

-       1 cup ice

DIRECTIONS

1. In a blender place all ingredients and blend until smooth

2. Pour smoothie in a glass and serve

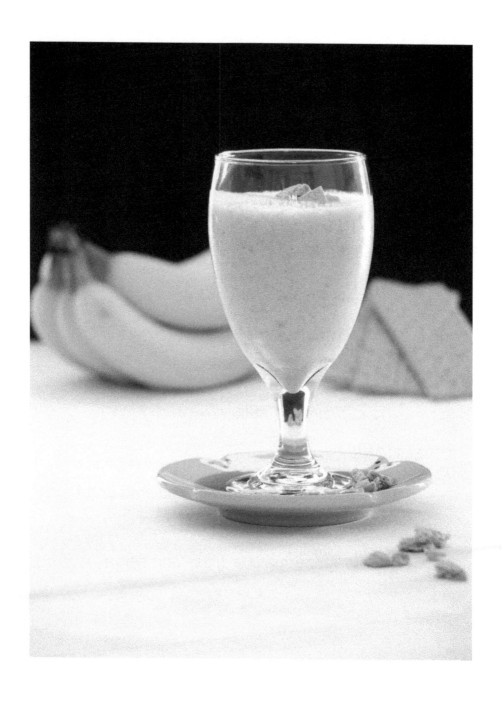

BERRY SMOOTHIE

Serves: *1*

Prep Time: *5*   Minutes

Cook Time: *5*   Minutes

Total Time: *10* Minutes

INGREDIENTS

- ¼ cup raspberries

- ½ cup strawberries

- 1 cup chocolate

- 1 cup almond milk

DIRECTIONS

1. In a blender place all ingredients and blend until smooth

2. Pour smoothie in a glass and serve

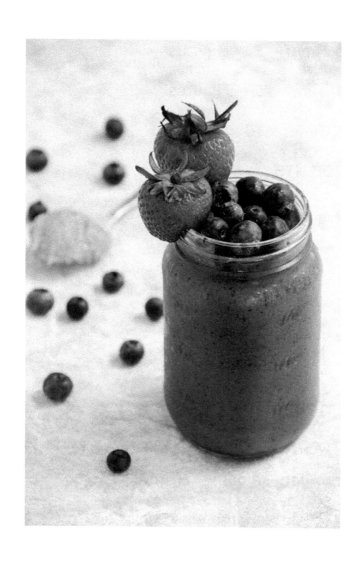

TROPICAL SMOOTHIE

Serves: *1*

Prep Time: *5* Minutes

Cook Time: *5* Minutes

Total Time: *10* Minutes

INGREDIENTS

- 1 cup pineapple

- ¼ banana

- 1 tsp vanilla essence

- ½ cup coconut milk

- 1 cup ice

DIRECTIONS

1. In a blender place all ingredients and blend until smooth

2. Pour smoothie in a glass and serve

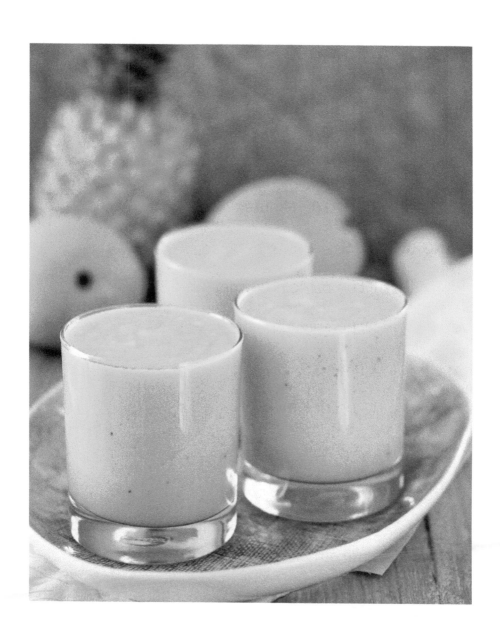

PROTEIN SMOOTHIE

Serves: *1*

Prep Time: *5*   Minutes

Cook Time: *5*   Minutes

Total Time: *10*   Minutes

INGREDIENTS

-        1 cup protein powder

-        1 cup spinach

-        1 pear

-        1 cup rice milk

-         1 cup ice

DIRECTIONS

1. In a blender place all ingredients and blend until smooth

2. Pour smoothie in a glass and serve

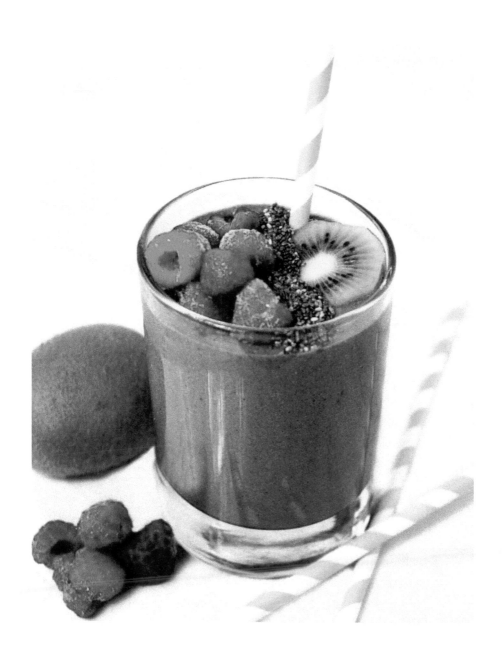

ORANGE SMOOTHIE

Serves: *1*

Prep Time: *5*   Minutes

Cook Time: *5*   Minutes

Total Time: *10*   Minutes

INGREDIENTS

- 2-3 carrots

- 1 stalk celery

- 1 cup pineapple

- ¼ lemon

- 1 orange

DIRECTIONS

1. In a blender place all ingredients and blend until smooth

2. Pour smoothie in a glass and serve

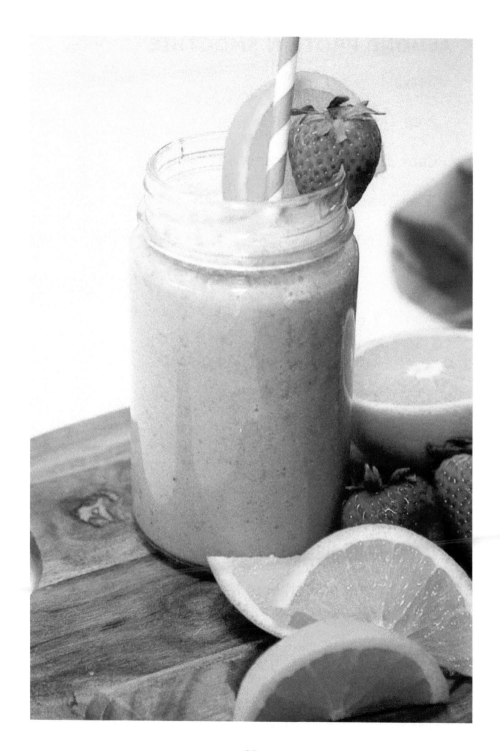

ALMOND PROTEIN SMOOTHIE

Serves: *1*

Prep Time: *5*   Minutes

Cook Time: *5*   Minutes

Total Time: *10*   Minutes

INGREDIENTS

-        1 cup protein powder

-        1 cup rice milk

-        1 tablespoon almond butter

-        1 banana

-        1 cup ice

DIRECTIONS

1. In a blender place all ingredients and blend until smooth

2. Pour smoothie in a glass and serve

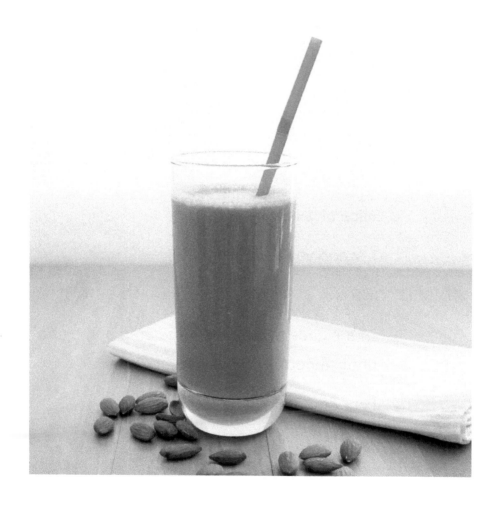

LEMON SMOOTHIE

Serves: 1

Prep Time: 5   Minutes

Cook Time: 5   Minutes

Total Time: 10   Minutes

INGREDIENTS

- 1 cup rice milk

- 1 cup blueberries

- Juice of 1 lemon

- 1 scoop vanilla powder

DIRECTIONS

1. In a blender place all ingredients and blend until smooth

2. Pour smoothie in a glass and serve

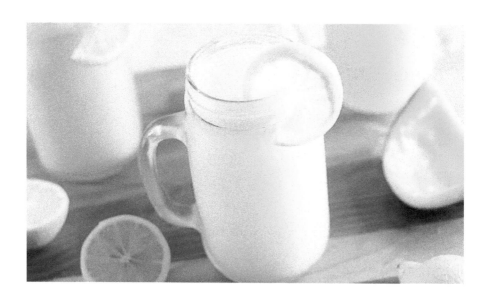

CHERRY SMOOTHIE

Serves: 1

Prep Time: 5   Minutes

Cook Time: 5   Minutes

Total Time: 10   Minutes

INGREDIENTS

-        1 cup almond milk

-        1 cup cherries

-        1 banana

-        1 scoop protein vanilla

DIRECTIONS

1. In a blender place all ingredients and blend until smooth

2. Pour smoothie in a glass and serve

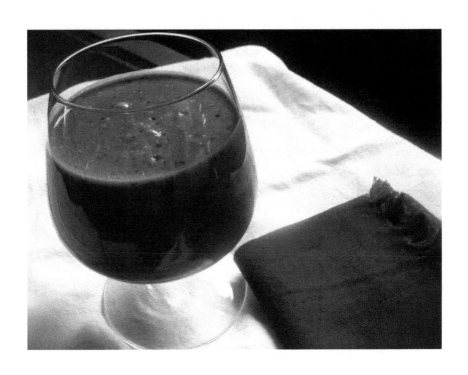

MANGO SMOOTHIE

Serves: *1*

Prep Time: *5*   Minutes

Cook Time: *5*   Minutes

Total Time: *10* Minutes

INGREDIENTS

-       1 mango

-       1 scoop protein powder

-       1 cup coconut milk

-       1 lime

-       1 cup ice

DIRECTIONS

1. In a blender place all ingredients and blend until smooth

2. Pour smoothie in a glass and serve

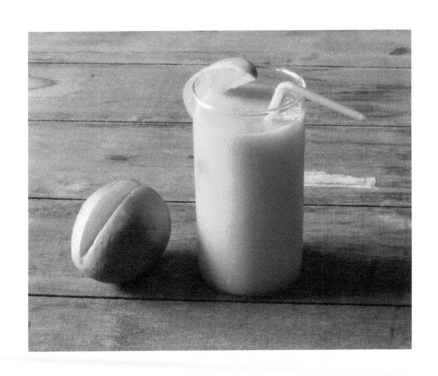

BAKED EGGS WITH VEGETABLE HASH

Serves: *2*

Prep Time: *10*   Minutes

Cook Time: *20*   Minutes

Total Time: *35*   Minutes

INGREDIENTS

- ¼ cup tomatoes

- ½ cup zucchini

- ½ cup yellow pepper

- 1 tablespoon olive oil

- 1 avocado

- 2 eggs

- salt

DIRECTIONS

1. Preheat the oven to 400 F

2. In a casserole dish add vegetables and drizzle olive oil over vegetables, mix well

3. Cut avocado in half, crack the eggs into each avocado half and sprinkle salt

4. Bake avocado and vegetables for 18-20 minutes or until vegetables are soft and eggs started to thicken

5. When ready remove from the oven and serve

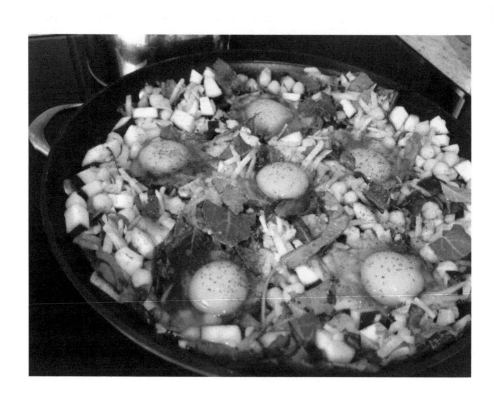

RUTABAGA HASH

Serves: 4

Prep Time: 10 Minutes

Cook Time: 20 Minutes

Total Time: 30 Minutes

INGREDIENTS

- 2 tablespoons olive oil

- 1 rutabaga

- ¼ cup red onion

- ¼ cup red pepper

- 1 tsp salt

- ¼ tsp pepper

- ¼ tsp dill

DIRECTIONS

1. In a skillet heat olive oil and sauté rutabaga for 4-5 minutes

2. Cover and cook until rutabagas are tender

3. Add red pepper, onion, paprika and sauté for 8-10 minutes

4. Add dill, pepper, salt and combine

5. When ready remove to a plate

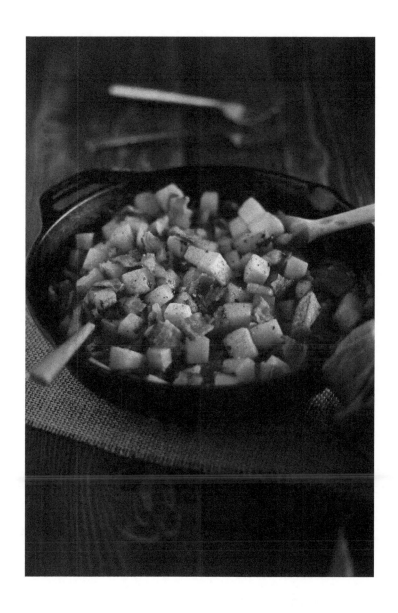

SAGE BREAKFAST PATTIES

Serves: *6*

Prep Time: *10*   Minutes

Cook Time: *15*   Minutes

Total Time: *25*   Minutes

INGREDIENTS

-        1 lb. turkey

-        1 tablespoon sage

-        1 tablespoon onions

-        ¼ tsp thyme

-        ¼ tsp garlic flakes

-        ¼ tsp salt

-        1 tablespoon olive oil

DIRECTIONS

1. In a bowl add all ingredients and mix well

2. Divide mixture into 4-6 portions and form 4-6 solid patties

3. In a skillet heat olive oil and cook each one for 4-5 minutes per side

4. When ready remove from skillet and serve

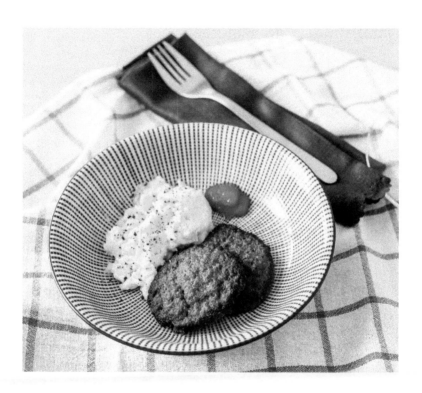

COCONUT CEREAL

Serves: *2*

Prep Time: *15* Minutes

Cook Time: *15* Minutes

Total Time: *30* Minutes

INGREDIENTS

- 1 cup almond flour

- ¼ tsp coconut

- 1 tsp cinnamon

- ¼ tsp salt

- ¼ tsp baking soda

- ¼ tsp vanilla extract

- 1 egg white

- 1 tablespoon olive oil

DIRECTIONS

1. Preheat the oven to 375 F

2. In a bowl combine baking soda, cinnamon, coconut, almond flour, salt and set aside

3. In another bowl combine vanilla extract, olive oil and mix well

4. In another bowl whisk the egg white and combine with vanilla extract mixture

5. Add almond flour to the vanilla extract mixture and mix well

6. Transfer dough onto a baking sheet and bake at 375 F for 10-15 minutes

7. When ready remove from the oven and serve

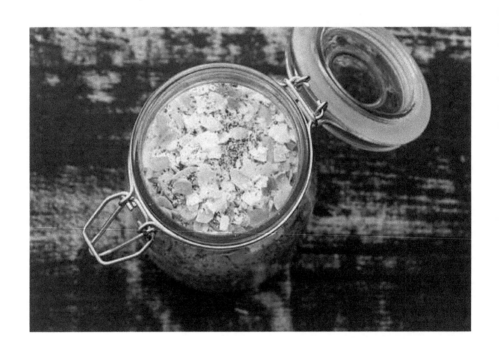

ZUCCHINI BREAD

Serves: *4*

Prep Time: *10* Minutes

Cook Time: *45* Minutes

Total Time: *55* Minutes

INGREDIENTS

- 1 zucchini

- 1 cup millet flour

- ½ cup almond flour

- ½ cup buckwheat flour

- 1 tsp baking powder

- ¼ tsp baking soda

- ¼ tsp salt

- ¼ cup almond milk

- 1 tsp apple cider vinegar

- 2 eggs

- ½ cup olive oil

DIRECTIONS

1. In a bowl combine almond flour, millet flour, buckwheat flour, baking soda, salt and mix well

2. In another bowl combine almond milk and apple cider vinegar

3. In a bowl beats eggs, add almond milk mixture and mix well

4. Add flour mixture to the almond mixture and mix well

5. Fold in zucchini and pour bread batter into pan

6. Bake at 375 F for 40-45 min

7. When ready remove from the oven and serve

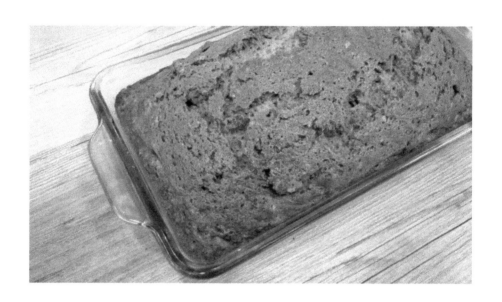

BAKED EGGS WITH ONIONS

Serves: *2*

Prep Time: *10*   Minutes

Cook Time: *20*   Minutes

Total Time: *30*   Minutes

INGREDIENTS

-         1 tablespoon olive oil

-         1 red bell pepper

-         1 red onion

-         1 cup tomatoes

-         ¼ tsp salt

-         ¼ tsp pepper

-         2 eggs

-         parsley

DIRECTIONS

1. In a saucepan heat olive oil and sauté peppers and onions until soft

2. Add salt, pepper, tomatoes and cook for 4-5 minutes

3. Remove mixture and form 2 patties

4. Break the eggs into each pattie, top with parsley and place under the broiler for 5-6 minutes

5. When ready remove and serve

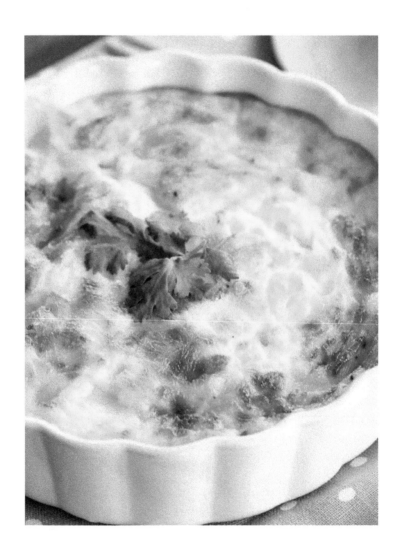

BIRCHER MUESLI

Serves: 2

Prep Time: 5 Minutes

Cook Time: 5 Minutes

Total Time: 10 Minutes

INGREDIENTS

- 1 cup coconut flakes

- ½ cup macadamia nuts

- 1 tablespoon chia seeds

- 1 tablespoon pumpkin seeds

- ¼ tsp cinnamon

- ¼ tsp ginger

- ¼ tsp nutmeg

DIRECTIONS

1. In a bowl combine all ingredients together

2. Place muesli in a container and refrigerate

3. When ready remove from the fridge and serve

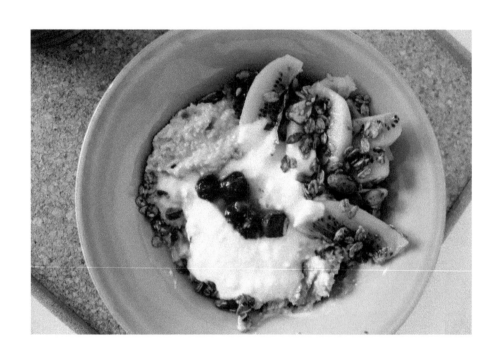

Lightning Source UK Ltd.
Milton Keynes UK
UKHW021013240621
386072UK00001B/83